BEYOND THE HIGHER POWER

I0102231

James T. Harman

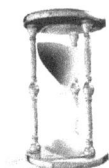

Prophecy
Countdown
Publications

BEYOND THE HIGHER POWER

Copyright © 1989, 2011, James T. Harman

Prophecy Countdown Publications
P.O. Box 941612
Maitland, FL 32794
www.ProphecyCountdown.com

Lightning Source
1246 Heil Quaker Blvd.
LaVergne, TN 37086
USA

First Edition – 1989
Second Edition – 2011
ISBN: 978-0-9636984-3-8

All references from Scripture are from the following sources:

NIV – Holy Bible, New International Version, copyright © 1973
LB – The Living Bible, copyright © 1971. Used by permission of
Tyndale House Publishers, Inc., Wheaton, IL 60189.
KJ – The King James Version, copyright © 1960

Words in bold emphasis are authors and not in original Scripture. Certain words are capitalized to emphasize their importance, but not in accordance with Traditional fashions.

Alcoholics Anonymous World Services, Inc. (AAWS) is not the source of this publication, and AAWS has not reviewed, approved or endorsed this publication or its contents or its source.

Dedication

This book is dedicated to the alcoholic or drug addict who is still struggling to get sober and wants to live a clean and purposeful life.

Higher Power

*"Let every soul be subject unto the **higher power**. For there is no power but of God: the powers that be are ordained of God."* (Romans 13:1 – KJ)

Table of Contents

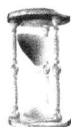

Preface

The purpose of this book is to relate an approach to dealing with alcohol and drugs that will help others find a new way of life. It is directed mainly at the alcoholic or drug addict who still suffers; but also will be of value to the person who is merely "dry" and not really free. Finally, it will be of interest to the sober alcoholic or other addicted person who wants to further develop the spiritual part of their individual program.

While many of the principles used in this book come from the program of Alcoholics Anonymous, it should be completely understood that it is not intended to be AA approved literature.

I want to say that I am indebted to the program of Alcoholics Anonymous and all the wonderful people who helped me in the very beginning to learn a new way of life. Without your care and love, I would not be writing this today.

Alcoholics Anonymous uses the twelve steps as the basis for the recovery program. These twelve steps originated from the Oxford Group's original ten steps. While these steps were based upon biblical teachings, most of the Christian basis was ignored when the twelve steps were written. This book will bring out the biblical basis upon which the steps were originally intended.

Jim Harman
3/17/1989

NOTES

Chapter 1 – You Are Not Alone

Hi, my name is Jim, and I'm an alcoholic. Today I say that I am an alcoholic with humility and a deep sense of gratitude that I found out what was wrong before it was too late.

For me to say that I am an alcoholic is something I never thought that I would be able to admit. I always thought of an alcoholic as someone on skid row. Everyone else knew that I had a problem with alcohol, but I sincerely didn't think that I was an alcoholic. I always thought that if only my ex-wife would change or if my job was only easier, then everything would be fine and I would be able to control my drinking. I would be able to "show them" that I was not an alcoholic.

As it turned out, "they" were right; but I was too stubborn to admit it. The real turning point came in my life when I HONESTLY admitted to myself that I had a problem and SINCERELY sought help. I got to the point where I was ready to take the first step.

STEP # 1
We admitted we were powerless over alcohol--that our lives had become unmanageable.

This first step is the hardest step for the alcoholic or drug addict to take. Throughout this book we will take a look at what the Bible has to say about our problem. There are several elements that the Bible helps us understand about ourselves:

Powerlessness
"You see, at just the right time, when we were still powerless, Christ died for the ungodly."
(Romans 5:6 – NIV)

"When we were utterly helpless with no way of escape, Christ came at just the right time and died for us sinners who had no use for him." (Romans 5:6 – LB)

The Bible clearly indicates that our position is one of complete powerlessness and helplessness. Until the alcoholic or drug addict is willing to admit this, there is little hope for recovery.

Competence
"Not that we are competent to claim anything for ourselves, but our competence comes from God." (II Corinthians 3:5 – NIV)

"Not because we think we can do anything of lasting value by ourselves. Our only power and success come from God." (II Corinthians 3:5 – LB)

Having realized that we are completely powerless and helpless, it is reassuring to know that there is someone that we can rely upon for our power and strength. Realizing that God wants to be our strength is one of the keys to overcoming our addiction.

Control
"I know that nothing good lives in me, that is, in my sinful nature. For I have the desire to do what is good, but I cannot carry it out. For what I do is not the good that I want to do; no, the evil I do not want to do--this I keep on doing. Now if I do what I do not want to do, it is no longer I who do it, but it is sin living in me that does it." (Romans 7:18-20 – NIV)

Once we realize that God wants to be our strength, we have to also understand what has been controlling our lives. As the above scripture indicates, the sin nature that we were born with is in control of our lives when we are drinking or doing drugs. I don't remember how many times that I tried to stop drinking.

I really wanted to stop, but was unable to. The problem was not only the drug, but also what the drug represented. That is, SIN. Sin was actually causing me to continue. Once the alcoholic or drug addict will recognize and admit that sin is the problem, they will be ready to receive help from the one that is the TRUE source.

True Vine

"I am the true vine and my Father is the gardner. He cuts off every branch in me that bears no fruit, while every branch that does bear fruit he trims clean so that it will be even more fruitful.

You are already clean because of the word I have spoken to you. Remain in me, and I will remain in you. No branch can bear fruit by itself; it must remain in the vine. Neither can you bear fruit unless you remain in me.

I am the vine; you are the branches. If a man remains in me and I in him, he will bear much fruit; apart from me you can do nothing." (John 15:1-5 – NIV)

In talking with his disciples, Jesus tells them that they can do nothing apart from him. Likewise as alcoholics or drug addicts, it is vital to come to the understanding of how completely helpless we are by ourselves.

But cheer up, you are not alone. There is hope in Jesus.

NOTES

Chapter 2 – Honesty And Acceptance

Once that first big step is made, it is important to come to a true understanding of who is capable of helping us. While the program of Alcoholics Anonymous talks about a *"power greater than ourselves"* or a *"higher power"*, the Bible is very clear as to the true source. The second step re-written from a biblical perspective might read:

STEP # 2
Came to believe that God through Jesus Christ alone can renew and restore us to soundness of mind and newness of life.

The Bible even indicates who the *"higher power"* is:

Higher Power
*"Let every soul be subject unto the **higher power**. For there is no power but of God: the powers that be are ordained of God."* (Romans 13:1 – KJ)

Included in the Old Testament is a story about a king who had to experience great loss before he was restored:

Sanity
"All this happened to King Nebuchadnezzar. Twelve months later, as the king was walking on the roof of the royal palace of Babylon, he said,"Is not this the great Babylon I have built by my mighty power and for the glory of my majesty?" The words were still on his lips when a voice came from heaven, "This is what is decreed for you, King Nebuchadnezzar: Your royal authority has been taken from you. You will be driven away from people and will live with the wild animals...
...(v33) .... immediately what had been said about

Nebuchadnezzar was fulfilled. He was driven away from people and ate grass like cattle (v34)...At the end of that time, I Nebuchadnezzar, RAISED MY EYES TOWARDS HEAVEN, AND MY SANITY WAS RESTORED, then I praised the Most High; I honored and glorified him who lives forever. (Daniel 4:28-34 – NIV)

This story parallels that of the alcoholic or drug addict. We have to receive the humility necessary in order to get us to look towards heaven. Once that is done, God can restore us. God is then ready to give us a new life:

New Life

"Therefore we are buried with him by baptism into death: ...as Christ was raised up from the dead by the glory of the Father, even so we also should walk in newness of life." (Romans 6:4 – KJ)

"I have been crucified with Christ and I no longer live, but Christ lives in me. The life I live in the body, I live by faith in the Son of God, who loved me and gave himself for me." (Galatians 2:20 – NIV)

"Therefore, if anyone is in Christ, he is a new creation; the old has gone, the new has come" (II Corinthians 5:17 – NIV)

The above scripture verses show that we really can have a new life! Once we DIE to our old way of living and ACCEPT Jesus Christ we become a brand new creation. This new life is available to anyone who HONESTLY wants to change and is willing to give their life completely to God.

Not only does God want to give us a brand new life, but he also wants to give us a sound mind:

Sound Mind

"For God hath not given us the spirit of fear; but of power, and of love, and of a sound mind."
(II Timothy 1:7 – KJ)

God wants to take away all fear from our lives. He wants us to have His power and love. He wants us to be a new creation, complete with a sound mind.

Once we are completely honest with ourselves and get to the stage in life that we are humble, God can give us a brand new life if we will only accept it. All He wants us to do is to enter into a new partnership with Him.

NOTES

Chapter 3 – A New Partnership

Having come to the point where we admit that we are completely powerless, and believe that God can help, we reach the crucial step:

> **Step # 3**
> Made a decision to turn our will and our lives over to the care of God through Jesus Christ.

This third step is the most important decision that the alcoholic or drug addict will ever make. It is essential to realize that we do not turn our life over merely to a *"God as we understood him."* While this concept is acceptable to people in general, it is not acceptable to God. Secular programs use this concept in order not to offend non-Christians.

This may make their program more popular, but it doesn't make it spiritually correct. The bible is quite clear on the way to know God:

Christ-Only Way
"I am the way and the truth and the life. No one comes to the Father except through me." (John 14:6 – NIV)

"...I tell you the truth, unless a man is born again, he cannot see the kingdom of God. "How can a man be born when he is old?" Nicodemus asked. "Surely he cannot enter a second time into his mother's womb to be born!"

Jesus answered, "I tell you the truth, unless a man is born of water AND the Spirit, he cannot enter the kingdom of God." (John 3:3-5 – NIV)

"...God has given us eternal life, and this life is in his Son, He who has the Son has life; he who does not have the Son of God does not have life."
(I John 5:11-12 – NIV)

"..for He longs for all to be saved and to understand this truth: That God is on one side and all the people on the other side, and Christ Jesus, himself man, is between them to bring them together, by giving his life for all mankind." (I Timothy 2:4-5 – LB)

God wants everyone to come to an understanding of who He is. He sent His only Son to give mankind a chance to truly live. Everyone is born a first time at child birth. Very few are actually born a second time, and unless a person is born by the Spirit of God, they will not see the Kingdom.

Having a knowledge of this is important. But knowing this without acting upon it does no good. Every alcoholic and drug addict who wants to overcome their addiction needs to act upon this information by making a decision:

Decision
"Now change your mind and attitude to God and turn to him so he can cleanse away your sins and send you wonderful times of refreshment from the presence of the Lord." (Acts 3:19 – NIV)

"Behold, I stand at the door, and knock: if any man hear my voice, and open the door, I will come in..."
(Revelation 3:20 – KJ)

"But to all who received him, to those who believed in his name, he gave the right to become children of God."
(John 1:12 – NIV)

God wants everyone to make the decision to turn to Him and
receive Jesus Christ into their heart. When we do this, God will
forgive all of our sins and cleanse us. We actually become a
child of God when we do this. After we open the door of our
heart and receive Jesus, He wants us to surrender our lives to
Him:

Surrendered Life

*"...Anyone who wants to follow me must put aside his
own desires and conveniences and carry his cross with
him every day and keep close to me."* (Luke 9:23 – LB)

*"I BESEECH you therefore, brethren, by the mercies of
God, that you present your bodies as a living sacrifice,
holy, acceptable unto God, which is your reasonable
service. And be not conformed to this world: but be
transformed by the renewing of your minds, that you
may prove what is that good, and acceptable, and
perfect will of God."* (Romans 12:1-2 – KJ)

God wants everyone to turn from their prior life of sin and live
each new day for Him. When we do this, God enters into a
partnership with you. He has a perfect will for each and every
person. All that He wants is your complete surrender to
Himself.

If you have never made a commitment to Jesus Christ before,
why not do so right now? Pray the following prayer:

*"Dear God, I know I am a sinner and I am unable to save
myself. But I do believe that You love me, and that You sent
Your Son Jesus, to die on the cross for all of my sins. Please
forgive my sins and give me the gift of eternal life. Please be the
Lord of my life and give me the gift of Your Holy Spirit, and
deliver me from the bondage of alcohol and drugs. Thank you
for hearing me and answering my prayer. In Jesus' name,
Amen."*

NOTES

Chapter 4 – Personal Housecleaning

If you prayed the prayer at the end of the last chapter, you have made the most important decision you will ever make in your life. You are now His child, and He will never leave you or forsake you.

After you have taken the first three steps, it is important to continue with the remaining steps. Only by continuing, can God make the changes in your life that are so necessary if you want to have the full and abundant life that He wants you to have.

The first thing you will need to do is some personal housecleaning:

Step # 4
Made a searching and fearless moral inventory of ourselves.

The purpose of this step is not to bring further condemnation upon ourselves, but to help us learn more about our personal assets and liabilities. First of all, it is important to realize that God already knows all about us:

God Sees All
"My eyes are on all their ways; they are not hidden from me, nor is their sin concealed from my eyes." (Jeremiah 16:17 – NIV)

"Can anyone hide in secret places so that 1 cannot see him? declares the Lord." Jeremiah 23:24 – NIV)

"His eyes are on the ways of men; he sees their every step." (Job 34: 21 – NIV)

"I obey your precepts and your statutes, for all my ways are known to you." (Psalm 119:168 – NIV)

"For a man's ways are in full view of the Lord, and he examines all his paths." (Proverbs 5:21 – NIV)

"O Lord, you have searched me and know me. You know when I sit and when I rise; you perceive my thoughts from afar. You discern my going out and my lying down; you are familiar with all my ways."
(Psalm 139:1-3 – N IV)

When you think about it, it is comforting to know that the God who created the universe takes such an intimate interest in each one of His children. God knows us better than we know ourselves. He wants us to examine our hearts with His help:

Search Heart
"Search me, O God, and know my heart; test me and know my anxious thoughts. See if there is any offensive way in me, and lead me in the way everlasting."
(Psalm 139:23-24 – NIV)

"For the word of God is living and active. Sharper than any double-edged sword, it penetrates even to dividing soul and spirit, joints and marrow; IT JUDGES THE THOUGHTS AND ATTITUDES OF THE HEART. Nothing in all creation is hidden from God's sight. Everything is uncovered and laid bare before the eyes of him to whom we must give account."
(Hebrews 4:12-13 – NIV)

God wants the recovering alcoholic or drug addict to begin a life of honestly searching their heart to examine underlying motives and attitudes. This fourth step is a lengthy exercise that requires complete honesty. Tools that will assist in taking this step include a good Bible and Hazelden's guide to the fourth step inventory.

Included in Appendix C, is a listing of the various character traits that should be examined when taking this step. The key is to ask God to give you an understanding about yourself. Pray for Him to show you the truth:

The Truth

"Jesus said to them, "If you continue in my word, then you are my disciples indeed; And you shall know the truth, and the truth shall make you free."
(John 8:31-32 – KJ)

If you will diligently seek the Lord by continuing to read His word on a daily basis, He will reveal the truth that you need to know about yourself. By prayer and daily bible study God will give us the insight into ourselves that will make us free.

NOTES

Chapter 5 – Cleansing

Having made a complete survey of our personal assets and our liabilities, we are ready for cleansing:

Step #5
Admitted to God, to ourselves and to another human being the exact nature of our wrongs.

As recovering alcoholics or drug addicts, it is important to know exactly what the bible has to say about sin:

Definitions of Sin

"Anyone, then, who knows the good he ought to do and doesn't do it sins." (James 4:17 – NIV)

"Everyone who sins breaks the law; in fact, sin is lawlessness. But you know that he appeared so that he might take away our sins." (I John 3: 4-5 – NIV)

"All wrongdoing is sin…" (I John 5:17 – NIV)

"Then David said to Nathan, "I have sinned against the Lord." (II Samuel 12:13 – NIV)

"Have mercy on me, 0 God, according to your unfailing love; according to your great compassion blot out my transgressions Wash away all my iniquity and cleanse me from my sin. For I know my transgressions, and my sin is always before me. Against you, you only, have I sinned and done what is evil in your sight, so that you are proved right when you speak and justified when you judge. Surely I have been a sinner since birth, sinful

from the time my mother conceived me. Surely you desire truth in the inner parts; you teach me wisdom in the inmost place.

Cleanse me with hyssop, and I will be clean; wash me, and I will be whiter than snow. Let me hear joy and gladness; let the bones you have crushed rejoice. Hide your face from my sins and blot out all my iniquity.

Create in me a pure heart, 0 God and renew a steadfast spirit within me. Do not cast me from your presence or take your Holy Spirit from me. Restore to me the joy of your salvation and grant me a willing spirit, to sustain me." (Psalm 51:1-12 – NIV)

David's prayer in the above Psalm shows why he was a man after God's own heart. David recognized that his sin was really against God and he asked God to cleanse and restore him. For a better understanding of the events which prompted this prayer, read II Samuel 11 and II Samuel 12:1-13.

After we have confessed our sins to God, the Bible instructs us to make confession to another person:

"He who conceals his sins does not prosper, but whoever confesses and renounces them finds mercy." (Proverbs 28:13 – NIV)

"Brothers, if someone is caught in a sin, you who are spiritual should restore him gently. But watch yourself, or you may also be tempted. Carry each other's burdens, and in this way you will fulfill the law of Christ." (Galatians 6:1-2 – NIV)

Notice that the Bible says to go to a "Brother". This means that the fifth step should be taken with another fellow believer in

Christ. The person selected should be a mature Christian that can be trusted.

Once we share our burdens with another, we are ready for the next two steps:

Step #6
Were entirely ready to have God remove all these defects of character.

Followed by:

Step #7
Humbly asked Him to remove our shortcomings.

These two steps are important for the alcoholic or drug addict to take in order to remove character defects and receive complete cleansing and healing.

Once the person becomes willing to acknowledge their sins and short comings, they are ready to take them to the Lord:

"Have mercy on me, O God, according to your unfailing love; according to your great compassion blot out my transgressions Wash away all my iniquity and cleanse me from my sin." (Psalm 51:1-2 – NIV)

"I sought the Lord, and he answered me; he delivered me from all my fears." (Psalm 34:4 – NIV)

"If we confess our sins, he is faithful and just and will forgive us our sins and purify us from all unrighteousness." (I John 1:9 – NIV)

God will forgive us, cleanse us, and deliver us. He wants to give us a new life that is free of all the sins of the past. These steps of cleansing make it possible for the alcoholic or drug addict to rid themselves of their past mistakes and sins, and walk in "newness of life" described in Romans 6:4:

> *"Therefore we are buried with him by baptism into death: that like as Christ was raised up from the dead by the glory of the Father, even so we also should walk in newness of life."* (Romans 6:4 – KJ)

> *"For we died and were buried with Christ by baptism. And just as Christ was raised from the dead by the glorious power of the Father, now we also may live new lives."* (Romans 6:4 – LB)

Through the process of cleansing and dying to our old way of living, God offers us brand new lives.

Chapter 6 – Reconciliation

After the alcoholic or drug addict has been reconciled to God, the next two steps should be taken in order to be reconciled with those who have been harmed:

Step #8
Made a list of all persons we had harmed, and became willing to make amends to them all.

Followed by:

Step #9
Made direct amends to such people wherever possible, except when to do so would injure them or others.

A list of those who have been harmed by past actions of the addicted person needs to be prepared with much care and prayer.

The Bible is quite clear that God wants people to be reconciled:

> "...if your brother sins, rebuke him, and if he repents, forgive him. If he sins against you seven times in a day, and seven times comes back to you and says, "I repent," forgive him." (Luke 17:3-4 – NIV)

> "Then Peter came to Jesus and asked, "Lord, how many times shall I forgive my brother when he sins against me? Up to seven times?" Jesus answered, "I tell you, not seven times, but seventy times seven times."
> (Matthew 18:21-22--NIV)

> "Do not repay anyone evil for evil. Be careful to do

what is right in the eyes of everybody. If it is possible, as far as it depends on you, live at peace with everyone." (Romans 12:17-18 – NIV)

"In your anger do not sin. Do not let the sun go down while you are still angry, and do not give the devil a foothold. He who has been stealing must steal no longer, but must work, doing something useful with his own hands, that he may have something to share with those in need. Do not let any unwholesome talk come out of your mouths, but only what is helpful for building others up according to their needs, that it may benefit those who listen. And do not grieve the Holy Spirit of God, with whom you were sealed for the day of redemption. Get rid of all bitterness, rage and anger, brawling and slander, along with every form of malice.

"Be kind and compassionate to one another, forgiving each other, just as in Christ God forgave you." (Ephesians 4:26-32 – NIV)

"For if you forgive men when they sin against you, your heavenly Father will also forgive you. But if you do not forgive men their sins, you Father will not forgive your sins." (Matthew 6:14-15--NIV)

Every attempt should be made to be reconciled with those who have been harmed by our past actions while drinking or doing drugs.

Not everyone will forgive, but it is the addicts job to attempt to be reconciled with everyone. There are, however, certain instances where this will be next to impossible. Some individuals may have been harmed to such a degree that they do not want to be reminded of the pain. In these cases it may be best to pray for those involved, but not attempt further confrontation.

The spirit of these steps is to make amends. God is concerned with our relationships, and He wants to mend them wherever possible.

NOTES

Chapter 7 – Repeated Examination

Having made reconciliation with God and others, the alcoholic or drug addict has made great strides in mending relationships.

In order to grow in these relationships, the addict needs to continue a daily self-examination of all attitudes and motives:

Step #10
Continued to take personal inventory and when we were wrong, promptly admitted it.

The Scripture verse relating to Step #4, is also appropriate for this step:

> *"Search me, O God, and know my heart; test me and know my anxious thoughts. See if there is any offensive way in me, and lead me in the way everlasting."*
> (Psalm 139:23-24 – NIV)

Also appropriate is:

> *"All a man's ways seem right to him, but the Lord weighs the heart."* (Proverb 21:2 – NIV)

The recovering alcoholic or drug addict will want to set aside a regular time each day to examine the motives of their heart. The Christian walk requires honesty and purity before the Lord. For God to even hear our prayers, we need to insure that our relationship with him is not broken due to our sin:

> *"If I had cherished sin in my heart, the Lord would not have listened; but God has surely listened and heard my voice in prayer. Praise be to God who has not rejected my prayer or withheld his love from me!"*
> (Psalm 66:18-19 – NIV)

"But your iniquities have separated you from you God; your sins have hidden his face from you, so that he will not hear." (Isaiah 59:2 – NIV)

"If anyone turns a deaf ear to the law, even his prayers are detestable." (Proverbs 28:9 – NIV)

For additional references that show how sin separates us from fellowship with God, please see: Jeremiah 11:11, Job 35:13, John 9:31, Zechariah 7:13, and Micah 3:4.

Finally, we have the assurance of God's word that when we confess our sins, He will forgive us:

"If we confess our sins, he is faithful and just and will forgive us our sins and purify us from all unrighteousness." (I John 1:9 – NIV)

To maintain a close relationship with God, we need to continually take our shortcomings before Him to ask for forgiveness.

Chapter 8 – Spiritual Growth

Having established a relationship with God, and maintaining it through a continual self-examination of the heart, the recovering addict is ready to cultivate that relationship through:

Step #11
Sought through prayer, study of His word, and meditation to know God and grow in constant contact with Him, praying only for knowledge of His will and the power to carry it out.

Prayer

The foundation for our relationship with God is prayer. Two acronyms that describe this activity are ACTS and PRAY:

Adoration	Praise
Confession	Repentance
Thanksgiving	Ask for others
Supplication	Yourself

Use either one or both of these acronyms to help focus during the time you spend in prayer.

The most popular prayer is the one Jesus taught us in Matthew 6:9-13 (NIV):

"Our Father in heaven, hallowed be your name, your kingdom come, your will be done on earth as it is in heaven. Give us today our daily bread. Forgive us our debts, as we also have forgiven our debtors. And lead us not into temptation, but deliver us from the evil one."

Entire books have been written on the Lord's prayer. Spending time before the Lord is the most important part of each day.

Study of His Word

While spending time with God in prayer, you will also want to spend time studying His word:

> *"...he is to read it (God's word) all the days of his life so that he may learn to revere the Lord his God and follow carefully all the words of this law and these decrees..."*
> (Deuteronomy 17:19 – NIV)

> *"Do your best to present yourself to God as one approved, a workman who does not need to be ashamed and who correctly handles the word of truth."*
> (II Timothy 2:15 – NIV)

> *"All Scripture is God-breathed and is useful for teaching, rebuking, correcting and training in righteousness so that the man of God may be thoroughly equipped for every good work."*
> (II Timothy 3:16-17 – NIV)

Meditation

In addition to spending time reading God's word to be equipped for service to the Lord, the recovering addict will want to spend time on a regular basis in meditation with Him:

> *"Do not let this Book of the Law depart from your mouth; meditate on it day and night, so that you may be careful to do everything written in it. Then you will be prosperous and successful."* (Joshua 1:8 – NIV)

> *"But his delight is in the law of the Lord, and on his law he MEDITATES day and night."* (Psalm 1:2 – NIV)

Wisdom & Knowledge

The word of God promises to be a rich storehouse:

"...turning your ear to wisdom and applying your heart to understanding, and if you callout for insight and cry aloud for understanding, and if you look for it as for silver and search for it as for hidden treasure, then you will understand the fear of the Lord and find the knowledge of God." (Proverbs 2:2-5 – NIV)

"Get wisdom, get understanding; do not forget my words or swerve from them." (Proverbs 4:5 – NIV)

God's Will
Diligently seeking God and His Word, leads to a knowledge of His will for our lives:

"I desire to do your will, 0 my God; your law is within my heart." (Psalm 40:8 – NIV)

"Teach me to do your will, for you are my God; may your good Spirit lead me on level ground." (Psalm 143:10 – NIV)

"Thy kingdom come. Thy will be done in earth, as it is in heaven." (Matthew 6:10 – KJ)

"What you ought to say is, "IF THE LORD WANTS US TO, we shall live and do this or that." James 4:15 – LB)

"How can a young man keep his way pure? By living according to your WORD. I seek you with all my heart; do not let me stray from your commands. I have hidden your word in my heart that I might not sin against you ...(v.11) ...I MEDITATE on your precepts and consider your ways. I delight in your decrees; I will not neglect your word... (v.15-16)... Open my eyes that I may see wonderful things in your law... (v.18)...your servant will meditate on your decrees. Your statutes are my delight;

they are my counselors." (Psalm 119:9-24 – NIV)

"For I know the plans I have for you," declares the Lord, "plans to prosper you and not to harm you, ·plans to give you hope and a future. Then you will call upon me and come and pray to me, and I will listen to you. You will SEEK ME and FIND ME when you SEEK ME with ALL YOUR HEART." (Jeremiah 29:11-13 – NIV)

What wonderful promises God has in-store for anyone who will seek Him with all of their heart. God wants us to spend time with Him on a continual basis. By prayer, study of His Word, and meditation we can know God and His will for our life. God promises to prosper us and give us success when we diligently work this step.

Chapter 9 – Continual Service

Once an individual has honestly and sincerely attempted to work the preceding steps, the final step is a natural continuation that is born out of the new found way of life. It is with a deep sense of joy and gratitude that most will feel when taking this final step:

Step #12
Having had a spiritual awakening as a result of these steps, we tried to carry this message to other alcoholics and addicts, and to practice these principles in all our affairs.

This step can be broken into several parts:

Comfort others
"Praise be to the God and Father of our Lord Jesus Christ,...who comforts us in all our troubles, so that we can comfort those in any trouble with the comfort we ourselves have received from God."
(II Corinthians 1:3-4 – NIV)

Since the alcoholic or drug addict has found a new way of life practicing the first eleven steps, they will want to share their experiences so others can find similar success. Remember, it is by giving away that we truly receive.

Be Reconciled
"All this is from God, who reconciled us to himself through Christ and gave us the ministry of reconciliation: that God was reconciling the world to himself in Christ, not counting men's sins against them. And he has committed to us the message of reconciliation. We are therefore Christ's ambassadors,

as though God were making his appeal through us. We implore you on Christ's behalf: Be reconciled to God."
(II Corinthians 5: 18-20 – NIV)

Restoration
"Brothers, if someone is caught in sin, you who are spiritual should restore him gently..."
(Galatians 6:1 – NIV)

God wants to enlist the services of His new recruits to carry the message to those who are still in bondage in order for them to be reconciled and restored.

Teach others
"For you must teach others those things you and many others have heard me speak about. Teach these great truths to trustworthy men who will, in turn, pass them on to others." (II Timothy 2:2 – LB)

In order for the message to be continued, God wants reliable men and women to teach others. In this way, the message is passed on from generation to generation and people are helped in the process.

Fish for Men
"Come, follow me," Jesus said, "and I will make you fishers of men." (Matthew 4:19 – NIV)

Jesus was speaking to fishermen, but his statement is just as appropriate to the recovering alcoholic or drug addict that has been changed by a personal encounter with Him.

Make Disciples
"Therefore go and make disciples of all nations, baptizing them in the name of the Father and of the Son and of the Holy Spirit, and teaching them to obey

everything I have commanded you. And surely I will be with you always, to the very end of the age. "
(Matthew 28:19-20 – NIV)

Becoming a follower of Jesus Christ requires commitment and discipline. Jesus' promise to be with us should give us the courage to carry out His assignment. In addition, there is another promise found in Hebrews 6:10 (NIV) that should be an encouragement:

> *"God is not unjust; he will not forget your work and the love you have shown him as you have helped his people and continue to help them."*

Working the twelve steps eventually becomes a way of life. The recovering alcoholic or drug addict will find a joy and peace in their life that they have never known and that they never thought possible.

Because of this, they will want to share this wonderful message with those who still suffer.

NOTES

Appendix A – Twelve Steps to Recovery

1. I ADMIT I NEED HELP
We admitted we were powerless over alcohol--that our lives had become unmanageable.

2. I BELIEVE GOD CAN HELP
Came to believe that God through Jesus Christ alone can renew and restore us to soundness of mind and newness of life.

3. I DECIDE FOR GOD
Made a decision to turn our will and our lives over to the care of God through Jesus Christ.

4. I LOOK AT MYSELF
Made a searching and fearless moral inventory of ourselves.

5. I CONFESS MY WRONGS
Admitted to God, to ourselves and to another human being the exact nature of our wrongs.

6. I AM READY TO BE CHANGED
Were entirely ready to have God remove all these defects of character.

7. I ASK GOD TO HELP
Humbly asked Him to remove our shortcomings.

8. I THINK OF THOSE I HAVE HARMED
Made a list of all persons we had harmed, and became willing to make amends to them all.

9. I MAKE AMENDS
Made direct amends to such people wherever possible, except when to do so would injure them or others.

Appendix A Twelve Steps to Recovery (Continued)

10. I CONTINUE TO LOOK AT MYSELF
Continued to take personal inventory and when we were wrong, promptly admitted it.

11. I DRAW CLOSER TO GOD
Sought through prayer, study of His Word, and meditation to know God and grow in constant contact with Him, praying only for knowledge of His Will and the power to carry it out.

12. I HELP OTHERS
Having had a spiritual awakening as a result of these steps, we tried to carry this message to other alcoholics and addicts, and to practice these principles in all our affairs.

Appendix B – A Personal Invitation

Working the twelve steps as outlined in this book will change the life of the alcoholic, drug addict, or other addicted person. One of the key steps to this new way of life is discussed in the third chapter, "A New Partnership."

If you have never made a commitment to Jesus Christ before, why not do so right now? Pray the following prayer:

> *"Dear God, I know I am a sinner and I am unable to save myself. But I do believe that You love me, and that You sent Your Son Jesus, to die on the cross for all of my sins. Please forgive my sins and give me the gift of eternal life. Please be the Lord of my life and give me the gift of Your Holy Spirit, and deliver me from the bondage of alcohol and drugs. Thank you for hearing me and answering my prayer. In Jesus' name, Amen."*

Signed_____

Date_____

"For I know the plans I have for you," declares the LORD, "plans to prosper you and not to harm you, plans to give you hope and a future. Then you will call upon me and come and pray to me, and I will listen to you. You will seek me and find me when you seek me with all your heart." (Jeremiah 29:11-13 – NIV)

"Search me, O God, and know my heart: try me, and know my thoughts" (Psalm 139:23 – KJ)

"Search me, O God, and know my heart; test me and know my anxious thoughts. See if there is any offensive way in me, and lead me in the way everlasting." (Psalm 139:23-24 – NIV)

"Jesus said to them, "If you continue in my word, then you are my disciples indeed; And you shall know the truth, and the truth shall make you free." (John 8:31-32 – KJ)

Appendix C – Personal Inventory

The following pages list the various character traits that the recovering alcoholic or drug addict should examine when taking the fourth and tenth steps. Useful tools that should be used in conjunction with this appendix include: the Bible and Hazelden's guide to the fourth step inventory.

For convenience, the liability and asset of each common trait are listed on facing pages.

Liability	Asset	Pages
Pride	Humility	48-49
Envy	Generosity	50-51
Perfectionism	Admitting Mistakes	52-53
Being Phony	Being Yourself	54-55
Selfishness	Sharing	56-57
Self-Pity	Serenity	58-59
Impatience	Patience	60-61
Intolerance	Tolerance	62-63
Alibis	Being Honest	64-65
Dishonest Thinking	Honesty	66-67
Procrastination	Perseverance	68-69
Guilt Feelings	Freedom from Guilt	70-71
Resentment	Forgiveness	72-73
Fear	Faith	74-75
Hate	Love	76-77

Jesus taught us that we are to love God and our neighbor as ourselves. Alcoholics and drug addicts need to learn how to properly love themselves. An honest personal assessment of your assets and liabilities is an essential step in learning to have a healthy self-love that will enable you to love others. Use the following pages to make an honest examination of yourself.

PERSONAL INVENTORY

PRIDE
An overly high opinion of oneself.

Personal Analysis:

_____

_____

_____

_____

_____

_____

_____

_____

_____

_____

_____

_____

_____

_____

_____

_____

_____

_____

PERSONAL INVENTORY

HUMILITY
Accepting ones strengths and weaknesses without trying to justify them.

Personal Analysis:

_____

_____

_____

_____

_____

_____

_____

_____

_____

_____

_____

_____

_____

_____

_____

_____

_____

_____

_____

PERSONAL INVENTORY

ENVY
Excessive desire of possessions of others.

Personal Analysis:

_____

_____

_____

_____

_____

_____

_____

_____

_____

_____

_____

_____

_____

_____

_____

_____

_____

_____

_____

_____

_____

PERSONAL INVENTORY

GENEROSITY
Capable of giving and sharing freely.

Personal Analysis:

_____

_____

_____

_____

_____

_____

_____

_____

_____

_____

_____

_____

_____

_____

_____

_____

_____

_____

_____

PERSONAL INVENTORY

PERFECTIONISM
Setting unrealistically high standards and unwilling to accept mistakes.

Personal Analysis:

_____

_____

_____

_____

_____

_____

_____

_____

_____

_____

_____

_____

_____

_____

_____

_____

_____

_____

_____

PERSONAL INVENTORY

ADMITTING MISTAKES
Accepting mistakes as part of being human.

Personal Analysis:

_____

_____

_____

_____

_____

_____

_____

_____

_____

_____

_____

_____

_____

_____

_____

_____

_____

_____

_____

PERSONAL INVENTORY

BEING PHONY
Trying to impress others or make them think higher of oneself.

Personal Analysis:

_____

_____

_____

_____

_____

_____

_____

_____

_____

_____

_____

_____

_____

_____

_____

_____

_____

_____

_____

_____

PERSONAL INVENTORY

BEING YOURSELF
Not worrying about what others think. Being transparent.

Personal Analysis:

_____

_____

_____

_____

_____

_____

_____

_____

_____

_____

_____

_____

_____

_____

_____

_____

_____

_____

_____

_____

PERSONAL INVENTORY

SELFISHNESS
Thinking of oneself before others.

Personal Analysis:

_____

_____

_____

_____

_____

_____

_____

_____

_____

_____

_____

_____

_____

_____

_____

_____

_____

_____

_____

_____

PERSONAL INVENTORY

SHARING
Being able to give of oneself.

Personal Analysis:

_____

_____

_____

_____

_____

_____

_____

_____

_____

_____

_____

_____

_____

_____

_____

_____

_____

_____

_____

PERSONAL INVENTORY

SELF-PITY
Feeling sorry for oneself.

Personal Analysis:

_____

_____

_____

_____

_____

_____

_____

_____

_____

_____

_____

_____

_____

_____

_____

_____

_____

_____

_____

_____

PERSONAL INVENTORY

SERENITY
Acceptance through centering on others instead of oneself.

Personal Analysis:

_____

_____

_____

_____

_____

_____

_____

_____

_____

_____

_____

_____

_____

_____

_____

_____

_____

_____

_____

PERSONAL INVENTORY

IMPATIENCE
Unwillingness to wait.

Personal Analysis:

_____

_____

_____

_____

_____

_____

_____

_____

_____

_____

_____

_____

_____

_____

_____

_____

_____

_____

_____

PERSONAL INVENTORY

PATIENCE
Being tolerant, forbearing. Uncomplaining endurance.

Personal Analysis:

_____

_____

_____

_____

_____

_____

_____

_____

_____

_____

_____

_____

_____

_____

_____

_____

_____

_____

_____

_____

PERSONAL INVENTORY

INTOLERANCE
Refusal to tolerate others.

Personal Analysis:

_____

_____

_____

_____

_____

_____

_____

_____

_____

_____

_____

_____

_____

_____

_____

_____

_____

_____

_____

PERSONAL INVENTORY

TOLERANCE
Ability to see and accept other points of view.

Personal Analysis:

_____

_____

_____

_____

_____

_____

_____

_____

_____

_____

_____

_____

_____

_____

_____

_____

_____

_____

_____

_____

PERSONAL INVENTORY

ALIBIS
Self-justification of ones behavior through excuses.

Personal Analysis:

_____

_____

_____

_____

_____

_____

_____

_____

_____

_____

_____

_____

_____

_____

_____

_____

_____

_____

_____

_____

PERSONAL INVENTORY

BEING HONEST
Sincere and truthful with oneself and others.

Personal Analysis:

_____

_____

_____

_____

_____

_____

_____

_____

_____

_____

_____

_____

_____

_____

_____

_____

_____

_____

_____

_____

PERSONAL INVENTORY

DISHONEST THINKING
Another way of lying.

Personal Analysis:

_____

_____

_____

_____

_____

_____

_____

_____

_____

_____

_____

_____

_____

_____

_____

_____

_____

_____

_____

_____

_____

PERSONAL INVENTORY

HONESTY
Being truthful, open and frank. Being genuine.

Personal Analysis:

_____

_____

_____

_____

_____

_____

_____

_____

_____

_____

_____

_____

_____

_____

_____

_____

_____

_____

_____

_____

PERSONAL INVENTORY

PROCRASTINATION
Putting things off until the last minute.

Personal Analysis:

_____

_____

_____

_____

_____

_____

_____

_____

_____

_____

_____

_____

_____

_____

_____

_____

_____

_____

_____

_____

PERSONAL INVENTORY

PERSEVERANCE
Steadfast adherence to achieve desired goal.

Personal Analysis:

_____

_____

_____

_____

_____

_____

_____

_____

_____

_____

_____

_____

_____

_____

_____

_____

_____

_____

_____

_____

PERSONAL INVENTORY

GUILT FEELINGS
False guilt about the past.

Personal Analysis:

_____

_____

_____

_____

_____

_____

_____

_____

_____

_____

_____

_____

_____

_____

_____

_____

_____

_____

_____

_____

PERSONAL INVENTORY

FREEDOM FROM GUILT
Believing that God will forgive once we repent.

Personal Analysis:

_____

_____

_____

_____

_____

_____

_____

_____

_____

_____

_____

_____

_____

_____

_____

_____

_____

_____

_____

PERSONAL INVENTORY

RESENTMENT
Feeling of bitterness, anger and hatred towards others.

Personal Analysis:

_____

_____

_____

_____

_____

_____

_____

_____

_____

_____

_____

_____

_____

_____

_____

_____

_____

_____

_____

_____

PERSONAL INVENTORY

FORGIVENESS
Accepting others when wronged.

Personal Analysis:

_____

_____

_____

_____

_____

_____

_____

_____

_____

_____

_____

_____

_____

_____

_____

_____

_____

_____

_____

PERSONAL INVENTORY

FEAR
Expectation of bad consequences in the future.

Personal Analysis:

_____

_____

_____

_____

_____

_____

_____

_____

_____

_____

_____

_____

_____

_____

_____

_____

_____

_____

_____

_____

_____

_____

PERSONAL INVENTORY

FAITH
Confident assurance of God's care.

Personal Analysis:

_____

_____

_____

_____

_____

_____

_____

_____

_____

_____

_____

_____

_____

_____

_____

_____

_____

_____

_____

_____

PERSONAL INVENTORY

HATE
Intense animosity.

Personal Analysis:

_____

_____

_____

_____

_____

_____

_____

_____

_____

_____

_____

_____

_____

_____

_____

_____

_____

_____

_____

_____

_____

PERSONAL INVENTORY

LOVE
Sacrificial choice that seeks the highest and best for the person who is the object of that love.

Personal Analysis:

_____

_____

_____

_____

_____

_____

_____

_____

_____

_____

_____

_____

_____

_____

_____

_____

_____

_____

_____

_____

_____

NOTES

Appendix D – What the Bible Says About It

Included on the following pages are excerpts from the Bible on various topics listed below that will be of interest to the recovering alcoholic or drug addict.

Appendix D – WHAT THE BIBLE SAYS ABOUT IT:

ONE DAY AT A TIME

"However, if you do not obey the Lord your God and do not carefully follow all his commands and decrees I am giving you today, all these curses will come upon you and overtake you: ....In the morning you will say, "If only it were evening!" and in the evening, "If only it were morning!"
(Deuteronomy 28:15 & 67 – NIV)

"So don't be anxious about tomorrow. God will take care of your tomorrow too. Live one day at a time."
(Matthew 6:34 – LB)

EASY DOES IT

"Come to me, all you who are weary and burdened, and I will give you rest. Take my yoke upon you and learn from me, for I am gentle and humble in heart, and you will find rest for your souls. For my yoke is easy and my burden is light."
(Matthew 11:28-30 – NIV)

"Peace I leave with you; my peace I give you. I do not give to you as the world gives. Do not let your hearts be troubled and do not be afraid." (John 14:27- NIV)

"He gives strength to the weary and increases the power of the weak." (Isaiah 40:29 – NIV)

"So do not fear, for I am with you; do not be dismayed, for I am your God. I will strengthen you and help you; I will uphold you with my righteous right hand." (Isaiah 41:10 – NIV)

"...because we have sought the Lord our God; we sought him and he has given us rest on every side."
(II Chronicles 14:7--NIV)

EASY DOES °IT (CONTINUED)
"He makes me lie down in green pastures, he leads me beside quiet waters..." (Psalm 23:2 – NIV)

BUT FOR THE GRACE OF GOD
"For the Lord God is a sun and shield; the Lord bestows favor and honor; no good thing does he withhold from those whose walk is blameless." (Psalm 84:11 – NIV)

"But you are a chosen people, a royal priesthood, a holy nation, a people belonging to God, that you may declare the praises of him who called you out of darkness into his wonderful light. Once you were not a people, but now you are the people of God; once you had not received mercy, but now you have received mercy." (I Peter 2:9-10 – NIV)

KEEP IT SIMPLE
"But I fear, lest by any means, as the serpent (Satan) beguiled Eve through his subtlety, so your minds should be corrupted from the SIMPLICITY that is in Christ."
(II Corinthians 11:3 – KJ)

FIRST THINGS FIRST
"Anyone who loves his father or mother more than me is not worthy of me; anyone who loves his son or daughter more than me is not worthy of me; and anyone who does not take his cross and follow me is not worthy of me. Whoever finds his life will loose it, and whoever loses his life for my sake will find it."
(Matthew 10:37-39 – NIV)

"As Jesus and his disciples were on their way, he came to a village where a woman named Martha opened her home to him. She had a sister named Mary, who sat at the Lord's feet LISTENING to what he said. But Martha was distracted by all the preparations that had to be made. She came to him and asked, "Lord, don't you care that my sister has left me to do the

work by myself? Tell her to help me!" "Martha, Martha," the Lord answered, "you are worried and upset about many things, but ONLY ONE THING is needed. Mary has chosen what is better, and it will not be taken away from her."
(Luke 10:38-42 – NIV)

"But seek FIRST his kingdom and his righteousness, and all these things will be given to you as well." (Matthew 6:33 – NIV)

LIVE AND LET LIVE

"Do not judge, or you too will be judged. For in the same way you judge others, you will be judged, and with the measure you use, it will be measured to you. Why do you look at the speck of sawdust in your brother's eye and pay no attention to the plank in your own eye? How can you say to your brother, 'Let me take the speck out of your eye,' when all the time there is a plank in your own eye? You hypocrite, first take the plank out of your own eye, and then you will see clearly to remove the speck from your brother's eye." (Matthew 7:1-5 – NIV)

"You, therefore, have no excuse, you who pass judgement on someone else, for at whatever point you judge the other, you are condemning yourself, because you who pass judgment do the same things." (Romans 2:1 – NIV)

"Therefore let us stop passing judgement on one another. Instead, make up your mind not to put any stumbling block or obstacle in your brother's way." (Romans 14:13 – NIV)

"Make it your ambition to lead a quiet life, to mind your own business and to work with your hands, just as we told you...."
(I Thessalonians 4:11 – NIV)

SPONSORS

"Brothers, if someone is caught in a sin, YOU WHO ARE SPIRITUAL should restore him gently....Carry each other's burdens, and in this way you will fulfill the law of Christ."
(Galatians 6:1-2 – NIV)

FEAR – FAITH

"Do not be anxious about anything, but in everything, by prayer and petition, with thanksgiving, present your requests to God. And the peace of God, which transcends all understanding, will guard your hearts and your minds in Christ Jesus."
(Philippians 4;6-7 – NIV)

"So do not fear, for I am with you; do not be dismayed, for I am your God. I will strengthen you and help you; I will uphold you with my righteous right hand." (Isaiah 41:10 – NIV)

"He will have no fear of bad news; his heart is steadfast, trusting in the Lord. His heart is secure, he will have no fear; in the end he will look in triumph on his foes."
(Psalm 112:7-8 – NIV)

RESENTMENT (ANGER)

"In your anger do not sin:... Do not let the sun go down while you are still angry, and do not give the devil a foothold."
(Ephesians 4:26-27 – NIV)

"My dear brothers, take note of this: Everyone should be quick to listen, slow to speak and slow to become angry, for man's anger does not bring about the righteous life that God desires."
(James 1:19-20 – NIV)

GRATITUDE

"Let the word of Christ dwell in you richly as you teach and admonish one another with all wisdom, and as you sing psalms, hymns and spiritual songs with gratitude in your hearts to God..

...And whatever you do, whether in word or deed, do it all in the name of the Lord Jesus, giving thanks to God the Father through him. " (Colossians 3:16-17 – NIV)

SELF PITY

"When the sun rose, God provided a scorching east wind, and the sun blazed on Jonah's head so that he grew faint. He wanted to die, and said, "It would be better for me to die than to live." But God said to Jonah, "Do you have a right to be angry about the vine?" "I do," he said. "I am angry enough to die." But the Lord said, "You have been concerned about this vine, though you did not tend it or make· it grow. It sprang up overnight and died overnight. But Nineveh has more than a hundred and twenty thousand people who cannot tell their right hand from their left, and many cattle as well. Should I not be concerned about that great city?" (Jonah 4:8-11 – NIV)

IF

"Now listen, you who say, "Today or tomorrow we will go to this or that city, spend a year there, carry on business and make money." Why, you do not even know what will happen tomorrow. What is your life? You are a mist that appears for a little while and then vanishes. Instead, you ought to say, "IF it is the Lord's will, we will live and do this or that."
(James 4:13-15 – NIV)

SELFISHNESS

"For everyone looks out for his own interests, not those of Jesus Christ." (Philippians 2:21 – NIV)

"For I was hungry and you gave me nothing to eat, I was thirsty and you gave me nothing to drink..." (Matthew 25:42 – NIV)

"Suppose a brother or sister is without clothes and daily food. If

one of you says to him, "Go, I wish you well; keep warm and well fed," but does nothing about his physical needs, what good is it?" (James 2:15-16 – NIV)

"Nobody should seek his own good, but the good of others." (I Corinthians 10:24 – NIV)

PROBLEMS
"No temptation (problem) has seized you except what is common to man. And God is faithful; he will not let you be tempted beyond what you can bear. But when you are tempted, he will also provide a way out so that you can stand up under it." (I Corinthians 10:13 – NIV)

EGO
"For whoever exalts himself will be humbled, and whoever humbles himself will be exalted." (Matthew 23:12 – NIV)

"For in his own eyes he flatters himself too much to detect or hate his sin." (Psalm 36:2 – NIV)

"If anyone thinks he is something when he is nothing, he deceives himself." (Galatians 6:3 – NIV)

"This is the one I esteem: he who is humble and contrite in spirit..." (Isaiah 66:2 – NIV)

An acronym for ego is:

> Easing
> God
> Out

LOVE
"Love is patient, love is kind. It does not envy, it does not boast, it is not proud. It is not rude, it is not self-seeking, it is not

easily angered, it keeps no record of wrong. Love does not delight in evil but rejoices with the truth. It always protects, always trusts, always hopes, always perseveres. Love never fails. But where there are prophecies, they will cease; where there are tongues, they will be stilled; where there is knowledge, it will pass away. For we know in part and we prophecy in part, but when perfection comes, the imperfect disappears. When I was a child, I talked like a child, I thought like a child, I reasoned like a child. When I became a man, I put childish ways behind me. Now we see but a poor reflection; then we shall see face to face. Now I know in part; then I shall know fully, even as I am fully known. And now these three remain: faith, hope and Love. But the greatest of these is Love." (I Corinthians 13:4-13 – NIV)

LET GO and LET GOD
"Cast all your anxiety on him because he cares for you." (I Peter 5:7 – NIV)

"Trust in the Lord with all your heart and Lean not on your own understanding; in all your ways acknowledge him, and he will make your paths straight." (Proverbs 3:5-6 – NIV)

SERENITY PRAYER
"God, grant me the serenity to accept the things I can not change, The courage to change the things that I can, and The wisdom to know the difference." Anonymous

BIBLE
The following acronym is quite simple, but quite true and profound:

> Basic
> Instructions
> Before
> Leaving
> Earth

OVERCOMERS

"He who has an ear, let him hear what the Spirit says to the churches. To him who OVERCOMES, I will give the right to eat from the tree of life, which is in the paradise of God." (Revelation 2:7 – NIV)

"He who has an ear, let him hear what the Spirit says to the churches. To him who OVERCOMES, I will give some of the hidden manna. I will also give him a white stone with a new name written on it, known only to him who receives it." (Revelation 2:17 – NIV)

"To him who OVERCOMES and does my will to the end, I will give authority over the nations." (Revelation 2:26 – NIV)

"He who OVERCOMES will, like them, be dressed in white. I will never, erase his name from the book of life, but will acknowledge his name before my Father and his angels." (Revelation 3:5 – NIV)

"Him who OVERCOMES I will make a pillar in the temple of my God. Never again will he leave it. I will write on him the name of my God and the name of the city of my God, the new Jerusalem, which is coming down out of heaven from my God; and I will also write on him my new name." (Revelation 3:12 – NIV)

"To him who OVERCOMES, I will give the right to sit with me on my throne, just as I overcame and sat down with my Father on his throne." (Revelation 3:21 – NIV)

"They OVERCAME him by the blood of the Lamb and by the word of their testimony; they did not love their lives so much as to shrink from death." (Revelation 12:11 – NIV)

For more on being an Overcomer, please see our free book: **THE KINGDOM** available at: www.ProphecyCountdown.com

NOTES

Appendix E

Sign of Christ's Coming

April 8, 1997

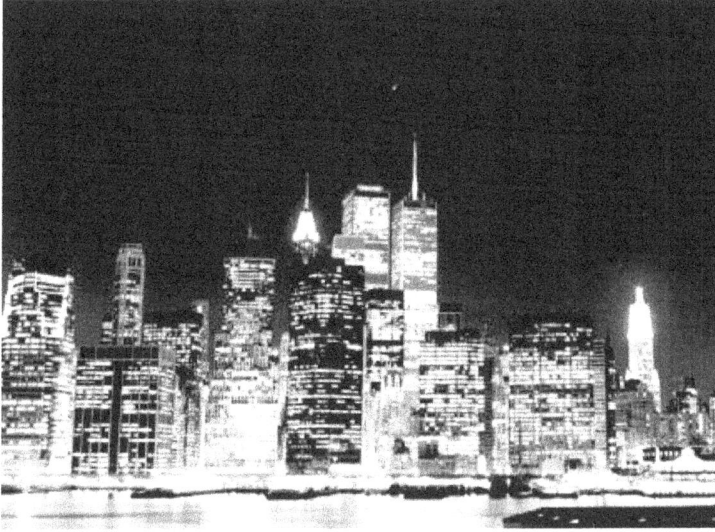

Comet Hale-Bopp Over New York City
Credit and Copyright: J. Sivo
http://antwrp.gsfc.nasa.gov/apod/ap970408.html

"What's that point of light above the World Trade Center? It's Comet Hale-Bopp! Both faster than a speeding bullet and able to "leap" tall buildings in its single underline orbit, Comet Hale-Bopp is also bright enough to be seen even over the glowing lights of one of the world's premier cities. In the foreground lies the East River, while much of New York City's Lower Manhattan can be seen between the river and the comet."

- -

"As it was in the days of Noah, so it will be at the coming of the Son of Man." (Matthew 24:37 – NIV)

These words from our wonderful Lord have several applications about the Tribulation period that is about to ensnare this world.

Seas Lifted Up
Throughout the Old Testament, the time of the coming Tribulation period is described as the time when the "seas have lifted up," and also as coming in as a "flood" (please see Jeremiah 51:42, Hosea 5:10, Daniel 11:40 and Psalm 93:3-4 for just a few examples).

This is a direct parallel to the time of Noah when the Great Flood of water came to wipe out every living creature except for righteous Noah and his family, and the pairs of animals God spared. While God said He would never flood the earth again with water, the coming Judgement will be by fire (II Peter 3:10). The book of Revelation shows that approximately three billion people will perish in the terrible time that lies ahead (see Revelation 6:8 and 9:15).

2 Witnesses
A guiding principle of God is to establish a matter based upon the witness of two or more:

> *"...a matter must be established by the testimony of two or three witnesses"* (Deuteronomy 19:15 – NIV)

In 1994, God was able to get the attention of mankind when Comet Shoemaker-Levy crashed into Jupiter on the 9th of Av (on the Jewish calendar). Interestingly, this Comet was named after the "two" witnesses who first discovered it.

In 1995, "two" more astronomers also discovered another comet. It was called Comet Hale-Bopp, and it reached its closest approach to planet Earth on March 23, 1997. It has been labeled as the most widely viewed comet in the history of mankind.

Scientists have determined that Comet Hale-Bopp's orbit brought it to our solar system 4,465 years ago (see Notes 1 and 2 below). In other words, the comet made its appearance near Earth in 1997 and also in 2468 BC. Remarkably, this comet preceded the Great Flood by 120 years! God warned Noah of this in Genesis 6:3:

> *"My Spirit shall not strive with man forever, for he is indeed flesh; yet his days shall be one hundred and twenty years."*

Days of Noah
What does all of this have to do with the Lord's return? Noah was born around 2948 BC, and Genesis 7:11, tells us that the Flood took place when Noah was 600, or in 2348 BC.

Remember, our Lord told us: *"As it was in the days of Noah, so it will be at the coming of the Son of Man."* (Matthew 24:37 – NIV)

In the original Greek, it is saying: *"exactly like"* it was, so it will be when He comes (see Strong's #5618).

During the days of Noah, Comet Hale-Bopp arrived on the scene as a harbinger of the Great Flood. Just as this same comet appeared before the Flood, could its arrival again in 1997 be a sign that God's final Judgement, also known as the time of Jacob's Trouble, is about to begin?

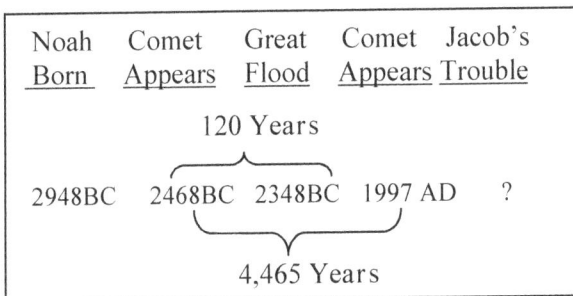

Noah Born	Comet Appears	Great Flood	Comet Appears	Jacob's Trouble
	120 Years			
2948BC	2468BC	2348BC	1997 AD	?
	4,465 Years			

Comet Hale-Bopp's arrived 120 years before the Flood as a warning to mankind. Only righteous Noah heeded God's warning and built the ark, as God instructed. By faith, Noah was obedient to God and, as a result, saved himself and his family from destruction.

Remember, Jesus told us His return would be preceded by great heavenly signs: *"And there shall be signs in the sun, and in the moon, and in the stars; and upon the earth distress of nations, with perplexity; the sea and the waves roaring..."* (Luke 21:25)

Just as this large comet appeared as a 120-year warning to Noah, its arrival in 1997 tells us that Jesus is getting ready to return again. Is this the **"Sign"** Jesus referred to?

> Jesus was asked 3 questions by the disciples:
> *"Tell us, (1) when shall these things be"* (the destruction of the city of Jerusalem), *" and (2) what shall be the __sign__ of thy coming, and (3) of the end of the world?"* (Matthew 24:3)

Sign of Christ's Coming

The **first** question had to do with events that were fulfilled in 70 AD. The **third** question has to do with the future time at the very end of the age.

The **second** question, however, has to do with the time of Christ's second coming. Jesus answered this second question in His description of the days of Noah found in Matthew 24:33-39:

(33) *"So likewise ye, when ye shall see all these things, know that it is near, even at the doors. (34) Verily I say unto you, This generation shall not pass, till all these things be fulfilled. (35) Heaven and earth shall pass away, but my words shall not pass away. (36) But of that day and hour knoweth no man, no, not the angels of heaven, but my Father only. (37)* **But as the days of Noe were, so shall also the coming of the Son**

of man be. *(38)For as in the days that were before the flood they were eating and drinking, marrying and giving in marriage, until the day that Noe entered into the ark, (39) And knew not until the flood came, and took them all away; so shall also the coming of the Son of man be."*

Jesus is telling us that the **sign** of His coming will be as it was during the days of Noah. As Comet Hale-Bopp was a sign to the people in Noah's day, its arrival in 1997 is a sign that Jesus is coming back again soon. Comet Hale-Bopp could be the very sign Jesus was referring to, which would announce His return for His faithful.

Remember, Jesus said, *"exactly as it was in the days of Noah, so will it be when He returns."* The appearance of Comet Hale-Bopp in 1997 is a strong indication that the Tribulation period is about to begin, but before then, Jesus is coming for His Bride!

Keep looking up! Jesus is coming again very soon!
As Noah prepared for the destruction God warned him about 120 years before the Flood, Jesus has given mankind a final warning that the Tribulation period is about to begin. The horrible destruction on 9/11 is only a precursor of what is about to take place on planet Earth. We need to be wise like Noah and prepare. Always remember our Lord's instructions:

Watch and Pray

*"(34)And take heed to yourselves, lest at any time your hearts be overcharged with surfeiting, and drunkenness, and cares of this life, and so that day come upon you unawares. (35) For as a snare shall it come on all them that dwell on the face of the whole earth. (36) **Watch ye therefore, and pray always, that ye may be accounted worthy to escape all these things that shall come to pass, and to stand before the Son of man"*** (Luke 21:34-36).

Footnotes

(1) The original orbit of Comet Hale-Bopp was calculated to be approximately 265 years by engineer George Sanctuary in his article: ***Three Craters In Israel***, published on March 31, 2001 that can be found at:
 http://www.gsanctuary.com/3craters.html#3c_r13

Comet Hale-Bopp's orbit around the time of the Flood changed from 265 years to about 4,200 years. Because the plane of the comet's orbit is perpendicular to the earth's orbital plane (ecliptic), Mr. Sanctuary noted: "A negative time increment was used for this simulation...to back the comet away from the earth.... past Jupiter... and then out of the solar system. The simulation suggests that the past-past orbit had a very eccentric orbit with a period of only 265 years. When the comet passed Jupiter (***around 2203BC***) its orbit was deflected upward, coming down near the earth 15 months later with the comet's period changed from 265 years to about (***4,200***) years." (***added text*** *for clarity*)

(2) Don Yeomans, with NASA's Jet Propulsion Laboratory made the following observations regarding the comet's orbit: "By integrating the above orbit forward and backward in time until the comet leaves the planetary system and then referring the osculating orbital elements...the following orbital periods result:
Original orbital period before entering planetary system = 4200 years. Future orbital period after exiting planetary system = 2380 years."
This analysis can be found at:
http://www2.jpl.nasa.gov/comet/ephemjpl6.html

Based upon the above two calculations we have the following:
265 [a] + 4,200 [b] = 4,465 Years
1997 AD – 4,465 Years = 2468 BC = Hale Bopp arrived

(a) Orbit period calculated by George Sanctuary before deflection around 2203 BC.
(b) Orbit period calculated by Don Yeomans after 1997 visit.

Special Invitation

It is hoped this book will help people come to know Jesus Christ as their "Higher Power." If you have never been saved before, would you like to be saved? The Bible shows that it's simple to be saved...

- Realize you are a sinner.
  "As it is written, There is none righteous, no, not one:"
  (Romans 3:10)
  "... for there is no difference. For all have sinned, and come short of the glory of God;" (Romans 3:22-23)
- Realize you CAN NOT save yourself.
  "But we are all as an unclean thing, and all our righteousness are as filthy rags; ..." (Isaiah 64:6)
  "Not by works of righteousness which we have done, but according to his mercy he saved us, ..." (Titus 3:5)
- Realize that Jesus Christ died on the cross to pay for your sins.
  "Who his own self bare our sins in his own body on the tree, ..." (I Peter 2:24)
  "... Unto him that loved us, and washed us from our sins in his own blood," (Revelation 1:5)
- Simply by faith receive Jesus Christ as your personal Savior.
  "But as many as received him, to them gave he power to become the sons of God, even to them that believe on his name:" (John 1:12)
  " ...Sirs, what must I do to be saved? And they said, Believe on the Lord Jesus Christ, and thou shalt be saved, and thy house." (Acts 16:30-31)
  "...if you confess with your mouth, 'Jesus is Lord,' and believe in your heart God raised him from the dead, you will be saved." (Romans 10:9 – NIV)

WOULD YOU LIKE TO BE SAVED?

If you want to be saved, you can receive Jesus Christ right now by making the following confession of faith:

> Lord Jesus, I know that I am a sinner, and unless you save me, I am lost. I thank you for dying for me at Calvary. By faith I come to you now, Lord, the best way I know how, and ask you to save me. I believe that God raised you from the dead and acknowledge you as my personal Saviour.

If you believed on the Lord, this is the most important decision of your life. You are now saved by the precious blood of Jesus Christ, which was shed for you and your sins. Now that you have received Jesus as your personal Saviour, you will want to find a Church where you can be baptized as your first act of obedience, and where the word of God is taught so you can continue to grow in your faith. Ask the Holy Spirit to help you as you read the Bible to learn all that God has for your life.

Also, please see the Suggested Reading section that follows where you will find recommended books and websites that will help you on your wonderful journey.

Endtimes

The Bible indicates that we are living in the final days and Jesus Christ is getting ready to return very soon. This book was written to help people prepare for what lies ahead. The word of God indicates that the Tribulation Period is rapidly approaching and that the Antichrist is getting ready to emerge on the world scene.

Jesus promised His disciples that there is a way to escape the horrible time of testing and persecution that will soon devastate this planet. One of the purposes of this book is to help you get prepared so you will be ready when Jesus Christ returns.

Suggested Reading

Alcoholics Anonymous
World Services, Inc.
New York, NY

Living Sober
Alcoholics Anonymous
World Services, Inc.
New York, NY

12 Steps & 12 Traditions
Alcoholics Anonymous
World Services, Inc.
New York, NY

Dying For A Drink
Anderson Spickard
Word Books
Waco, Texas

The Taste of New Wine
Keith Miller
Word Books
Waco, Texas

Other Recommended Books and Websites:

The following books and websites are highly recommended for those who want to learn more about the deeper Truths found in the Scriptures:

The Open Door
by Lyn Mize   www.ffruits.org
Worthy of the Kingdom
by Tom Finley   www.seekersofchrist.org
Judgment Seat of Christ
by D.M. Panton   www.schoettlepublishing.com
Kingdom, Power & Glory
by Nancy Missler   www.kingshighway.org

NOTES

About The Author

Jim Harman is a recovering alcoholic who has been successfully working the steps outlined in this book for over 32 years. During his attempt to overcome his bondage to alcohol and drugs, he came to a biblical understanding of who the "Higher Power" is.

Since coming to know Jesus as his Lord and Saviour, God has shown him the scriptural background to the 12 step program that he learned in Alcoholics Anonymous. He has seen these steps work in such programs as "The New Wine Fellowship" and the "Overcomers" groups, both of which are programs to help the alcoholic or drug addict recover.

He is so convinced regarding the principles outlined in this book that he says: "*I guarantee that anyone who wants to recover from alcoholism or drug addiction will recover if they honestly work the 12 steps outlined in **Beyond the Higher Power***."

Beyond the Higher Power was Jim's first book written back in 1989. Since then, he has diligently studied the word of God with a particular emphasis on Prophecy. Jim has written several books and the four most essential titles are available at www.ProphecyCountdown.com: ***The Coming Spiritual Earthquake, Don't Be Left Behind, The Kingdom, and Beyond the Lake of Fire;*** which have been widely distributed around the world. These books encourage many to continue *"Looking"* for the Lord's soon return, and bring many to a saving knowledge of Jesus Christ.

Jim's professional experience includes being a Certified Public Accountant (CPA) and a Certified Property Manager (CPM). He has an extensive background in both public accounting and financial management with several well known national firms.

Jim has been fortunate to have been acquainted with several mature believers who understand and teach the deeper truths of the Bible. It is Jim's strong desire that many will come to realize the importance of seeking the Kingdom and seeking Christ's righteousness as we approach the soon return of our Lord and Saviour Jesus Christ.

The burden of his heart is to see many come to know the joy of Christ's triumph in their life as they become true overcomers; qualified and ready to rule and reign with Christ in the coming Kingdom.

Jim and his wife Cindy began the ministry of **Prophecy Countdown** back in 1989 to help prepare the Bride of Christ for the return of our wonderful Bridegroom. All of their newsletters and books have been written to encourage the believer in Christ and to force them to dig deep into the Word to see what the Lord is telling us. On the following pages you will find descriptions of several of Jim's books that are available on their website or at Amazon.com.

To contact the author for questions or to arrange for speaking engagements:

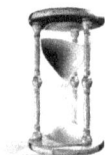

Jim Harman
P.O. Box 941612
Maitland, FL 32794
JimHarmanCPA@aol.com
www.ProphecyCountdown.com

*"And take heed to yourselves, lest at any time your hearts be overcharged with surfeiting, and drunkenness, and cares of this life, and so that day come upon you unawares. For like a snare shall it come on all them that dwell on the face of the whole earth. **Watch ye, therefore, and <u>pray always</u>, that ye may be <u>accounted worthy to escape</u> all these things that shall come to pass, and to stand before the Son of Man"*** (Luke 21:34-36).

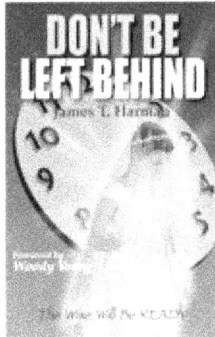

Is Daniel's Clock about to Start Ticking once again?
The recovery of the Old City of Jerusalem in June 1967 was a pivotal Prophetic Event. Find out how this major Prophetic Milestone may correlate with the start of the Second Half of Daniel's 70th Week.

> *"See to it that no one takes you captive through hollow and deceptive philosophy, which depends on human tradition and the basic principles of this world rather than on Christ."* (Colossians 2:8 NIV)

The "Traditional" teaching on the "70th Week of Daniel" has taken the Church captive into believing almost a "fairy tale" regarding Endtime events. Find out the beautiful Truth that has been hidden from modern day Christians.

MUST READING FOR EVERY CHRISTIAN

Jesus Christ is returning for His Bride. Are you "Watching" for your Bridegroom today? Find out the consequences of not being ready before the final grains of sand descend through the hour glass. Don't be one of those who will be LEFT BEHIND!

Order your copy today from www.ProphecyCountdown.com

Or from Amazon.com – Available in Paperback and or Kindle Edition

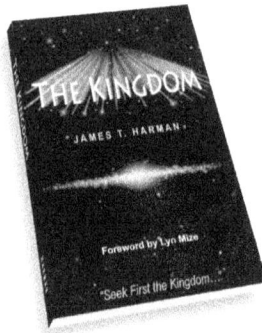

Once a person is saved, the number one priority should be seeking entrance into the Kingdom through the salvation of their soul. It is pictured as a runner in a race seeking a prize represented by a crown that will last forever.

The salvation of the soul and entrance into the coming Kingdom are only achieved through much testing and the trial of one's faith. If you are going through difficulty, then REJOICE:

> *"Blessed is the man who perseveres under trial, because when he has stood the test, he will receive the crown of life that God has promised to those who love Him."* (James 1:12)

The "Traditional" teaching on the "THE KINGDOM" has taken the Church captive into believing all Christians will rule and reign with Christ no matter if they have lived faithful and obedient lives, or if they have been slothful and disobedient with the talents God has given them. Find out the important Truth before Jesus Christ returns.

MUST READING FOR EVERY CHRISTIAN

Jesus Christ is returning for His faithful overcoming followers. Don't miss the opportunity of ruling and reigning with Christ in the coming KINGDOM!

Download your FREE copy: www.ProphecyCountdown.com

A poem about the virgins in Matthew 25:1-13

THE BRIDE – By Cindy Harman

A lamp with oil
All 10 did possess
But, remember, 5 were wise
And 5 were foolish.
Those who were wise
Heeded the call
By hearing God's voice:
"Give me your all"
The foolish however
Squandered their worth
They did not shine for Jesus
Nor the people on earth.
They heard "The Cry"
Along with the wise
This is how the foolish
Were taken by surprise:
Their light became impoverished
For their joy did not spread
The 'oil of gladness' for them
Flickered out instead.
But the wise grew brighter
With a special over-flow
The more they loved Jesus
They gained a purer glow.
Though the cry was mighty
Five questioned the call
They could not comprehend:
'Come give me your all.'
For if they truly loved Him
They would have understood the plea
For hidden in the message is:
'My Beloved come to Me.'
The 5 wise virgins heard this impassioned cry
....And answered 'Yes, my Beloved,
I am coming, it is I'
So they laid it all down
Living only to serve
The moral of the 10 virgins is:
Each got what they deserve.

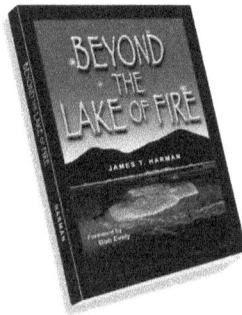

Go on a Journey back through the first 500 years of the Early Church to discover a teaching taught by Jesus and His Apostles. You will discover how one man emerged to change Church history forever – allowing Satan to create one of his greatest masterpieces.

> *"In whom the god of this world hath blinded the minds of them which believe not, lest the light of the glorious gospel of Christ, who is the image of God, should shine unto them."* (II Corinthians 4:4)

Learn what the "Glorious Gospel" really is and discover how God will use the Lake of Fire to restore mankind to the perfect state that existed before the fall of Adam.

The "Traditional" teaching on "Eternal Punishment" has captivated the Church with a belief that is contrary to what Jesus and the Apostles taught. Find out the important Truth before Christ returns.

Order your copy from Amazon.com – Available in Paperback

HELP DISTRIBUTE THIS MESSAGE

ARE YOU A WATCHMAN?
(Ezekiel 33:1-9)

Many people do not know the love God has for them in Christ. Help get this book to your friends and loved ones before Jesus returns very soon.

Prophecy Countdown Publications does not have the resources to distribute this important message to all the bookstores. Since we believe this information is so vital, this PDF book is being made available to everyone free of charge at: www.ProphecyCountdown.com. (See Tab called: *"Pastor's Corner"* Feel free to copy to your computer and e-mail to all those who you care about.

Order Extra Paperback Copies *

# of Copies	Total Costs (Includes Shipping & Handling)
1	$ 7
5	$ 25
10	$ 45
25	$100

*Order extra copies to give to friends and loved ones.

Please send check to: Jim Harman
                       P.O. Box 941612
                       Maitland, FL 32794

"The end of the age is coming soon. Therefore be earnest, thoughtful men of prayer."
(I Peter 4:7 – Paraphrase)

The Day of the Lord is Near!

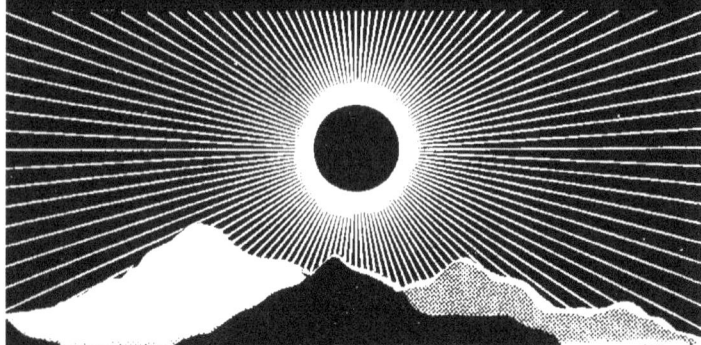

The Coming Spiritual Earthquake

by James T. Harman

"The Message presented in this book is greatly needed to awaken believers to the false ideas many have when it comes to the Rapture. I might have titled it: THE RAPTURE EARTHQUAKE!"
Ray Brubaker - God's News Behind the News

"If I am wrong, anyone who follows the directions given in this book will be better off spiritually. If I am right, they will be among the few to escape the greatest spiritual calamity of the ages."
Jim Harman - Author

**MUST READING FOR EVERY CHRISTIAN!
HURRY! BEFORE IT IS TOO LATE!**